LEUKEMIA DIET

Nourish, Heal, and Thrive – A
Comprehensive Guide to
Leukemia-Friendly Nutrition for
Enhanced Health and Recovery

Adams .U. Morris

TABLE OF CONTENTS

CHAPTER 1

leukemia diet

Leukemia is a formidable adversary, a complex group of blood cancers that impact the very core of our health - our blood and immune system. When one is diagnosed with leukemia, it can be a life-altering moment filled with fear and uncertainty. This book, "Leukemia Nutrition: Nourishing Your Journey to

Wellness," aims to shed light on an often-overlooked aspect of leukemia management - the role of nutrition.

Understanding Leukemia

Before we dive into the world of nutrition and its profound impact on leukemia, it's crucial to comprehend what leukemia is and how it affects the human body. Leukemia is a cancer that starts in the bone marrow, where blood cells are produced. Normally, the bone marrow produces healthy blood cells that are essential for various bodily functions, including transporting oxygen, fighting infections, and clotting to stop bleeding.

However, in leukemia, something goes awry in the bone marrow. It produces abnormal white blood cells, which are crucial components of our immune system. These abnormal cells do not function properly, and as they multiply uncontrollably, they can crowd out healthy blood cells. This leads to a compromised immune system, anemia (low red blood cell count), and an increased risk of bleeding (due to a low platelet count).

Importance of Nutrition in Leukemia Management

Leukemia, like many other cancers, is not just a disease that affects a single organ or system in the body. It has systemic effects, impacting not only the blood but also the organs and tissues that rely on healthy blood cells. Nutrition plays a pivotal role in managing leukemia for several reasons:

1. **Supporting the Immune System**: The immune system is a primary defense against cancer cells. Nutrients like vitamins, minerals, and antioxidants play a crucial role in maintaining a robust immune response. A well-nourished body is

better equipped to combat cancer cells and infections.

2. **Managing Treatment Side Effects**: Leukemia treatments, such as chemotherapy, radiation, and stem cell transplantation, can have harsh side effects. Proper nutrition can help mitigate these side effects, such as nausea, fatigue, and mouth sores, improving a patient's

quality of life during treatment.

3. **Maintaining Energy and Strength**: Leukemia can be physically taxing, causing fatigue and muscle weakness. Adequate nutrition ensures that the body has the energy and nutrients it needs to function optimally, even in the face of treatment-related challenges.

4. **Emotional Wellness**: Nutrition also plays a significant role in emotional well-being. Coping with leukemia can be mentally and emotionally draining. A nourishing diet can positively impact mood and overall mental health, aiding in the coping process.

Overview of the Book

In this book, we will take a deep dive into the world of

leukemia nutrition. We will explore not only the fundamentals of nutrition but also practical strategies and tips for tailoring your diet to your unique needs as a leukemia patient. You'll discover how to boost your immune system, manage treatment side effects, maintain energy and strength, and support your emotional well-being through mindful eating.

Each chapter is designed to be a stepping stone in your journey to wellness, offering insights, guidance, and practical advice. We'll provide you with a comprehensive understanding of the dietary considerations that can make a significant difference in your leukemia management and recovery.

The Personalized Approach to Nutrition

One of the key themes running through this book is

the importance of tailoring your diet to your specific needs. Leukemia is not a one-size-fits-all disease, and neither is nutrition. Every patient's journey is unique, influenced by factors such as the type of leukemia, its stage, and the individual's overall health.

Your leukemia may require a personalized nutrition plan, and that's where the guidance of a registered dietitian becomes invaluable. They can assess your dietary requirements, help you navigate the intricacies of nutrition during treatment, and provide you with a roadmap to better health.

It's important to recognize that what works for one leukemia patient may not work for another. By understanding your specific needs and making informed dietary choices, you can actively contribute to your well-being.

Real-Life Insights and Expert Perspectives

Throughout this book, we will draw upon the experiences of real-life leukemia patients who have successfully integrated nutrition into their treatment and recovery journey. These stories serve as beacons of hope, offering inspiration and practical insights into how nutrition can make a tangible difference.

We'll also tap into the expertise of oncologists and dietitians who have worked closely with leukemia patients. Their insights and recommendations are rooted in both scientific knowledge and the practical realities of managing leukemia through nutrition.

The Journey Ahead

As you embark on this journey through the pages of "Leukemia Nutrition: Nourishing Your Journey to

Wellness," remember that you are not alone. Leukemia is a formidable foe, but with the right knowledge, support, and determination, you can improve your quality of life and enhance your body's ability to fight this disease.

In the chapters that follow, we will delve deeper into the specific aspects of leukemia nutrition, offering practical advice, delicious recipes, and meal plans tailored to various stages of treatment and recovery. Whether you are a newly diagnosed patient, a caregiver, or a survivor seeking to maintain long-term wellness, this book is your guide to nourishing your journey to wellness.

CHAPTER 2

Understanding Leukemia

Leukemia is a complex and often bewildering condition, and in this chapter, we aim to shed light on its various aspects. To effectively navigate the path of leukemia management through nutrition, it's crucial to have a fundamental understanding of what leukemia is, how it affects the body, and what the different types and stages entail.

What is Leukemia?

Leukemia is a type of cancer that originates in the bone marrow and affects the blood and the immune system. To grasp its significance, we need to recognize the role of the bone marrow in our bodies. The bone marrow is like a biological factory responsible for producing three key types of blood cells: red blood cells

(RBCs), white blood cells (WBCs), and platelets.

- **Red Blood Cells (RBCs)**: These carry oxygen from the lungs to the rest of the body and return carbon dioxide to the lungs for exhalation. They are crucial for energy production and maintaining overall health.
- **White Blood Cells (WBCs)**: These are essential components of

the immune system, defending the body against infections and diseases. They are like the body's soldiers, constantly patrolling and guarding against invaders.

- **Platelets**: These are tiny cell fragments that help in blood clotting. When you get a cut, platelets rush to the site to stop the bleeding.

In leukemia, there is a mutation or change in the DNA of developing blood cells in the bone marrow. This mutation leads to the uncontrolled production of abnormal white blood cells. These abnormal cells, often referred to as leukemia cells, do not function properly. They multiply rapidly and can quickly outnumber the healthy blood cells.

Types and Stages of Leukemia

Leukemia is not a single disease but a group of related conditions, each with distinct characteristics. Two main categories classify leukemia:

1. **Acute Leukemia**: This type of leukemia progresses quickly, with the abnormal cells rapidly crowding out healthy blood cells. Acute leukemia is further divided into two main types: acute lymphoblastic leukemia

(ALL) and acute myeloid leukemia (AML). It is more common in children but can also occur in adults.

2. **Chronic Leukemia**: In contrast, chronic leukemia progresses more slowly, and the abnormal cells can still function somewhat normally. Chronic leukemia includes chronic lymphocytic leukemia (CLL) and chronic myeloid

leukemia (CML). It is more common in adults and often diagnosed during routine blood tests.

Understanding the type of leukemia is crucial because it determines the treatment approach and prognosis. Additionally, each type has further subtypes, making the landscape of leukemia highly diverse and complex.

Beyond the type, leukemia is also categorized into stages,

which describe the extent of the disease and how far it has spread. The stages typically range from 0 to IV, with 0 indicating an early stage and IV indicating an advanced stage. Staging helps guide treatment decisions and provides insight into the prognosis.

Impact on the Immune System

Leukemia's impact extends beyond the bone marrow. One of the most critical consequences is its effect on the immune system. The immune system is a complex network of cells, tissues, and organs that work together to defend the body against infections and diseases.

In a healthy individual, white blood cells play a pivotal role in immune function. They detect and destroy harmful pathogens like bacteria, viruses, and cancer cells. However, in leukemia, the bone marrow produces excessive numbers of abnormal white blood cells, often to the detriment of healthy ones. This imbalance compromises the immune system's ability to function effectively.

A weakened immune system means that leukemia patients are more susceptible to infections. Even minor illnesses that a healthy person might easily fight off can become serious threats. This heightened vulnerability underscores the importance of nutrition in leukemia management. A well-balanced diet that supports the immune system can be a potent ally in reducing the risk of infections and complications during treatment.

Common Symptoms and Side Effects

Leukemia often manifests with a range of symptoms, some of which can be subtle and easily dismissed, while others are more pronounced and alarming. Some common symptoms and side effects of leukemia include:

- **Fatigue**: Persistent and unexplained tiredness is a frequent complaint among leukemia patients. It can be caused by anemia (a low red blood cell count) or the leukemia cells themselves.

- **Bruising and Bleeding**: Low platelet counts can lead to easy bruising and prolonged bleeding even from minor cuts or injuries.

- **Frequent Infections**: A compromised immune system makes leukemia patients more susceptible to infections, resulting in recurrent illnesses.

- **Bone Pain**: Leukemia can cause pain in the bones and joints. This pain is often described as a deep, dull ache.

- **Swollen Lymph Nodes and Spleen**: Some leukemia types can cause the lymph nodes and spleen to enlarge, leading to discomfort or pain.
- **Weight Loss**: Unexplained weight loss can occur due to the body's increased energy demands and decreased appetite.
- **Fever**: Fever can be a sign of an infection,

which is more common in leukemia patients.

These symptoms can vary depending on the type and stage of leukemia. They can significantly impact a patient's quality of life and overall well-being. Managing these symptoms and side effects is an essential aspect of leukemia care and is where nutrition plays a crucial role.

In subsequent chapters of this book, we will delve deeper into how nutrition can be used to manage these side effects and enhance the overall quality of life for leukemia patients. We'll explore specific dietary strategies for supporting the immune system, addressing treatment-related challenges, and providing the body with the strength and energy it needs for the journey ahead.

Understanding leukemia's complexity, its impact on the immune system, and the symptoms and side effects it brings is the foundation upon which we will build our journey towards better nutrition and wellness. By gaining this knowledge, you are better equipped to make informed decisions about your dietary choices and how they can positively affect your leukemia management.

CHAPTER 3

Nutritional Basics

In our journey through leukemia management via nutrition, it's essential to start with the basics of nutrition itself. In this chapter, we'll explore the importance of a balanced diet and the key nutrients that are integral to supporting the body in its fight against leukemia. Let's embark on this foundational understanding of how food can be a powerful tool in your battle for wellness.

The Importance of a Balanced Diet

Nutrition is the cornerstone of our health. It provides the body with the necessary nutrients to function optimally, repair tissues, and maintain overall well-being. For leukemia patients, a balanced diet is not just a choice; it's a vital component of their treatment plan.

Here's why a balanced diet matters:

1. **Nutrient Supply**: A balanced diet ensures that the body receives all the essential nutrients it needs, including vitamins, minerals, carbohydrates, proteins, and fats. These nutrients are like the building blocks of life, playing roles in growth, immune function, energy production, and more.

2. **Immune Support**: Proper nutrition supports the immune system, which is of paramount importance for leukemia patients. White blood cells, a critical part of the immune system, depend on nutrients like vitamins A, C, D, and zinc to function effectively.

3. **Energy Production**: Fighting leukemia and undergoing treatment

can be physically demanding. A balanced diet provides the necessary calories and nutrients for energy, helping patients combat fatigue and maintain their strength.

4. **Tissue Repair**: Leukemia and its treatments can damage tissues in the body. Nutrients like protein, vitamin C, and zinc are essential for tissue repair and healing.

5. **Side Effect Management**: Certain nutrients can help manage treatment side effects. For example, a high-fiber diet can alleviate constipation, a common issue during treatment.

6. **Overall Well-Being**: Nutrition doesn't just impact the body; it affects mental and emotional health too. A well-balanced diet can

improve mood and overall quality of life.

Key Nutrients and Their Roles

Now, let's delve into some key nutrients and understand their specific roles in supporting the body during leukemia management:

1. **Proteins**: Proteins are crucial for cell repair and immune function. Leukemia patients may require more protein,

especially if they have undergone treatments like stem cell transplantation, which can lead to muscle loss. Sources of protein include lean meats, poultry, fish, eggs, dairy products, legumes, and tofu.

2. **Carbohydrates**: Carbohydrates are the body's primary energy source. Complex carbohydrates found in whole grains, fruits,

vegetables, and legumes provide sustained energy and fiber, which aids digestion and prevents constipation.

3. **Fats**: Healthy fats are essential for overall health and the absorption of fat-soluble vitamins (A, D, E, and K). Sources of healthy fats include avocados, nuts, seeds, and olive oil.

4. **Vitamins and Minerals**: Leukemia patients often have

increased nutrient needs due to the demands of treatment and the disease itself. Here are some key vitamins and minerals:

- **Vitamin C**: Boosts the immune system and aids in wound healing. Sources include citrus fruits, strawberries, and bell peppers.
- **Vitamin D**: Supports bone health and immune

function. Sunlight, fatty fish, and fortified foods are good sources.

- **Vitamin A:** Essential for immune function and skin health. Found in foods like carrots, sweet potatoes, and spinach.

- **Folate:** Supports cell division and repair. Sources include leafy greens, beans, and fortified cereals.

- **Calcium**: Important for bone health, especially if steroid medications are used. Dairy products, fortified plant-based milks, and leafy greens are sources.

- **Iron**: Helps prevent anemia, which can be a side effect of leukemia. Red meat, poultry, beans, and fortified cereals provide iron.

- **Zinc**: Supports immune function and wound healing. Foods like seafood, nuts, and whole grains are rich in zinc.

- **B vitamins**: Play various roles in metabolism, nerve function, and energy production. Whole grains, lean meats, and leafy greens are good sources.

5. **Fiber**: Dietary fiber aids in digestion and can alleviate constipation, a common issue for leukemia patients. It's found in fruits, vegetables, whole grains, and legumes.

6. **Fluids**: Staying hydrated is essential, especially during treatment, as it helps flush out toxins, supports

digestion, and prevents dehydration. Water, herbal teas, and clear broths are good options.

7. **Antioxidants**: These compounds, found in fruits and vegetables, protect cells from damage caused by free radicals and support overall health.

8. **Omega-3 Fatty Acids**: These healthy fats, found in fatty fish like salmon and in flaxseeds and walnuts, have anti-

inflammatory properties and support heart health.

Healthy Eating Guidelines for Leukemia Patients

Maintaining a healthy diet can be challenging during leukemia treatment, given the various side effects and symptoms. Here are some guidelines to help leukemia patients make informed dietary choices:

1. **Frequent, Small Meals**: Eating smaller,

more frequent meals can help manage nausea and prevent fatigue caused by large meals.

2. **Stay Hydrated**: Drink plenty of fluids, but avoid excessive caffeine and alcohol, which can contribute to dehydration.

3. **Choose Nutrient-Dense Foods**: Opt for foods rich in nutrients, as your body may have increased nutritional needs during treatment.

4. **Include Protein**:
Ensure an adequate
intake of protein to
support tissue repair and
immune function.

5. **Fiber-Rich Foods**:
Incorporate high-fiber
foods to aid digestion
and prevent
constipation.

6. **Limit Sugary Foods**:
Excessive sugar can
contribute to energy
fluctuations. Choose
natural sources of
sweetness like fruits.

7. **Moderate Salt**: High salt intake can lead to fluid retention. Use herbs and spices to flavor food instead.

8. **Consult a Registered Dietitian**: If you have specific dietary concerns or side effects, consider working with a registered dietitian who specializes in oncology nutrition. They can tailor a diet plan to your unique needs.

In subsequent chapters, we will explore how these nutritional basics can be applied practically to support the immune system, manage treatment side effects, maintain energy and strength, and promote emotional well-being throughout your leukemia journey. Understanding the role of nutrition and the importance of a balanced diet sets the stage for optimizing your health and quality of life as you navigate leukemia.

CHAPTER 4

Tailoring Your Diet to Your Needs

In the journey of leukemia management through nutrition, the concept of personalization takes center stage in Chapter 4. Here, we emphasize the critical importance of tailoring your diet to your specific needs as a leukemia patient. Each individual's experience with leukemia is unique, influenced by factors such as the type of leukemia, the stage of the disease, and the individual's overall health. This chapter aims to empower you with the knowledge and tools needed to make informed dietary choices that best suit your personal circumstances.

Why Personalization Matters

Leukemia is not a one-size-fits-all disease, and neither should be your approach to nutrition. Understanding the necessity for personalization is crucial for several reasons:

1. **Different Types of Leukemia**: As mentioned in earlier chapters, leukemia encompasses a range of types, including acute lymphoblastic leukemia (ALL), acute myeloid leukemia (AML), chronic lymphocytic leukemia (CLL), and chronic myeloid leukemia

(CML), among others. Each type may have different nutritional requirements based on how it affects the body.

2. **Staging Matters**: Leukemia is also staged to determine its extent and progression. The stage of the disease can significantly influence your nutritional needs and dietary recommendations. For example, a person with early-stage CLL may

have different dietary considerations than someone with advanced AML.

3. **Treatment Variation**: Leukemia treatment plans can vary widely. Some individuals may undergo chemotherapy, others may have stem cell transplantation, and treatment regimens may change over time. These treatments can impact your nutritional requirements and your

ability to tolerate certain foods.

4. **Overall Health**: Your overall health and any preexisting medical conditions also play a role in personalizing your diet. For example, if you have diabetes or heart disease in addition to leukemia, your dietary recommendations may need to address these conditions simultaneously.

Consulting a Registered Dietitian

One of the first steps in personalizing your diet as a leukemia patient is to consult a registered dietitian, ideally one with experience in oncology nutrition. These professionals have the expertise to assess your specific needs, taking into account your type of leukemia, its stage, and your overall health status.

During your consultation, the dietitian will:

- Conduct a comprehensive nutritional assessment to understand your dietary habits, preferences, and any challenges you may face.
- Evaluate your current nutritional status, including any nutrient deficiencies or excesses.
- Work with you to establish dietary goals

that align with your treatment plan and overall health objectives.

- Create a personalized nutrition plan that considers your unique circumstances and provides practical guidance on food choices and meal planning.

A registered dietitian can also serve as a valuable resource throughout your leukemia journey, offering ongoing support, monitoring, and adjustments to your nutrition plan as needed.

Specific Considerations for Personalization

Let's explore some specific areas where personalization plays a pivotal role in tailoring your diet to your needs:

1. **Dietary Restrictions**: Depending on your treatment and overall health, you may need to adhere to certain dietary restrictions. For

example, if you're on blood-thinning medications, you might need to limit foods high in vitamin K, which can interfere with these medications.

2. **Caloric Needs**: Personalization takes into account your caloric needs, which can vary greatly among leukemia patients. Factors like age, gender, activity level, and the stage of your disease

influence your daily calorie requirements.

3. **Nutrient Needs**: Based on your nutritional assessment, your dietitian will help you determine whether you need specific supplements or fortified foods to address nutrient deficiencies or ensure optimal intake of essential vitamins and minerals.

4. **Treatment-Related Challenges**: Different

leukemia treatments can present unique dietary challenges. For instance, if you're experiencing mouth sores or taste changes due to chemotherapy, your dietitian can recommend soft, bland foods that are easier to tolerate.

5. **Food Preferences and Allergies**: Personalization also takes into account your food preferences and any allergies or intolerances

you may have. This ensures that your nutrition plan is realistic and sustainable for you.

Maintaining a Balanced Diet

While personalization is key, it's essential to remember that the foundation of your diet should remain a balanced and nutritious one. Regardless of the specifics of your personalized plan, certain dietary principles hold true:

1. **Balanced Macronutrients**: Aim for a balance of carbohydrates, proteins, and fats to meet your energy needs and support overall health.

2. **Variety**: Incorporate a wide variety of foods to ensure a diverse intake of nutrients. Different foods provide different vitamins, minerals, and antioxidants.

3. **Hydration**: Stay adequately hydrated, as

it's crucial for overall health and can help manage treatment-related side effects.

4. **Fruits and Vegetables**: These should form a substantial part of your diet. They provide essential vitamins, minerals, fiber, and antioxidants.

5. **Portion Control**: Pay attention to portion sizes to avoid overeating or under-eating.

6. **Limit Processed Foods**: Minimize the consumption of highly processed and sugary foods, which offer little nutritional value.

7. **Moderation**: Enjoy treats and less nutritious foods in moderation, as long as they align with your dietary restrictions and don't compromise your overall health.

Monitoring and Adaptation

Your nutritional needs can change throughout your leukemia journey. Therefore, it's crucial to maintain regular communication with your healthcare team and dietitian. They can monitor your progress, adjust your nutrition plan as needed, and provide guidance to address any emerging challenges or side effects.

In the subsequent chapters of this book, we will delve deeper into specific aspects of leukemia nutrition, including immune system support, managing treatment side effects, maintaining energy and strength, and promoting emotional well-being. Personalization is the key to navigating these challenges effectively. By working closely with your healthcare team and making informed dietary choices, you can optimize your nutrition plan to enhance your quality of life and support your body as it battles leukemia.

CHAPTER 5

Eating to Boost Immunity

In Chapter 5, we dive into the crucial topic of boosting immunity through nutrition for leukemia patients. The immune system plays a pivotal role in the body's defense against cancer and infections, making it vital to ensure that it's operating at its best. We'll explore how specific nutrients and dietary choices can enhance your immune function, helping you better navigate the challenges of leukemia and its treatment.

The Immune System and Leukemia

Understanding the connection between the immune system and leukemia is fundamental. The immune system is like the body's defense army, responsible for identifying and eliminating harmful invaders, including cancer cells. In leukemia, where there's an overproduction of abnormal white blood cells (leukemia cells), the immune system can become overwhelmed or compromised.

Leukemia cells can crowd out healthy white blood cells, reducing the immune system's ability to function effectively. This makes leukemia patients more susceptible to infections and other health complications. However, through proper nutrition, you can give your immune system the support it needs to mount a robust defense.

Immune-Boosting Nutrients

Several key nutrients are known to play crucial roles in supporting and bolstering the immune system. Incorporating these nutrients into your diet can be particularly beneficial as a leukemia patient:

1. **Vitamin C:** This antioxidant vitamin is famous for its immune-boosting properties. It supports the production and function of white blood cells, which are integral to the immune response. Citrus fruits like oranges and grapefruits, as well as strawberries and bell peppers, are excellent sources of vitamin C.

2. **Vitamin D**: Vitamin D is essential for immune

function and can help your body fight infections. Exposure to sunlight is a natural way to synthesize vitamin D. Dietary sources include fatty fish (salmon, mackerel), fortified foods, and supplements if recommended by your healthcare team.

3. **Vitamin E:** This antioxidant vitamin plays a role in immune function and can help protect cells from

damage. Good sources include nuts, seeds, and spinach.

4. **Zinc**: Zinc is a mineral that's essential for immune cell development and function. Oysters, beef, beans, and nuts are rich sources of zinc.

5. **Protein**: Adequate protein intake is vital for the production and repair of immune cells. Lean meats, poultry, fish, dairy products, and

plant-based sources like beans and tofu can help you meet your protein needs.

6. **Beta-Carotene**: Beta-carotene is converted into vitamin A in the body, which is crucial for immune function. It's found in foods like carrots, sweet potatoes, and spinach.

7. **Selenium**: This trace element is involved in the production of enzymes that help

protect against infections. Brazil nuts, fish, and whole grains are good sources.

8. **Antioxidants**: Antioxidants like those found in berries, leafy greens, and other colorful fruits and vegetables help protect immune cells from damage caused by free radicals.

Immune-Boosting Foods

Incorporating immune-boosting foods into your diet is a practical way to support your immune system as a leukemia patient:

1. **Citrus Fruits**: Oranges, grapefruits, lemons, and limes are rich in vitamin C, a powerful immune booster.

2. **Berries**: Blueberries, strawberries, and raspberries are packed with antioxidants and

vitamins that enhance immune function.

3. **Garlic**: Garlic has antimicrobial and immune-enhancing properties. It's a flavorful addition to many dishes.

4. **Yogurt**: Probiotics found in yogurt can promote gut health, which is closely linked to immune function.

5. **Fatty Fish**: Salmon, mackerel, and trout are high in omega-3 fatty acids, which have anti-

inflammatory effects and support immune function.

6. **Nuts and Seeds**: Almonds, sunflower seeds, and hazelnuts are rich in vitamin E and zinc, both of which are vital for immune health.

7. **Leafy Greens**: Spinach, kale, and other leafy greens provide a wide array of vitamins and minerals, including vitamin A and folate,

which support immune function.

8. **Ginger and Turmeric**: These spices have anti-inflammatory and immune-boosting properties. They can be used in teas, soups, and various dishes.

Meal Planning for Immune Support

Crafting meals that prioritize immune support can be enjoyable and delicious. Here's how you can plan your meals to boost your immune system:

1. **Balanced Diet**: Ensure your meals include a balance of protein, carbohydrates, and healthy fats to provide overall nutrition.

2. **Colorful Plate**: Aim to have a variety of colorful fruits and vegetables on your plate, as different colors often represent different immune-

boosting antioxidants and nutrients.

3. **Incorporate Superfoods**: Superfoods like berries, nuts, seeds, and fatty fish can be regular additions to your diet.

4. **Hydration**: Stay well-hydrated, as dehydration can weaken your immune system. Herbal teas, water with lemon, and broths are excellent options.

5. **Probiotics**: Include probiotic-rich foods like yogurt or kefir to support gut health, which is closely linked to immune function.

6. **Limit Sugar and Processed Foods**: Excessive sugar and processed foods can weaken the immune system. Limit these items in your diet.

7. **Moderation**: While emphasizing immune-boosting foods,

remember that balance is key. Enjoy treats and less nutritious foods in moderation.

Supplements and Immunity

In some cases, your healthcare team may recommend specific supplements to support your immune system. This decision is typically based on your individual nutritional needs and the specifics of your leukemia and treatment. It's essential to consult with your healthcare provider before starting any supplements to ensure they are safe and appropriate for you.

In the subsequent chapters of this book, we will delve into additional aspects of leukemia nutrition, including managing treatment side effects, maintaining energy and strength, and promoting emotional well-being. As you explore the world of immune-boosting nutrition, remember that your dietary choices can be a powerful tool in enhancing your body's defenses against leukemia and infections, ultimately contributing to your overall well-being.

CHAPTER 6

Managing Treatment
Side Effects

Chapter 6 of "Leukemia Nutrition: Nourishing Your Journey to Wellness" delves into the critical topic of managing treatment side effects through diet. Leukemia treatments, which often include chemotherapy and radiation therapy, can bring about a host of physical challenges and discomforts. Proper nutrition can significantly alleviate these side effects, improve your overall quality of life, and support your body's ability to fight leukemia effectively.

Understanding Treatment Side Effects

Before we explore how nutrition can help manage treatment side effects, it's essential to understand the various challenges leukemia patients face during treatment. These side effects can vary depending on the type of leukemia, the stage, and the specific treatment regimen. Common treatment-related side effects include:

1. **Nausea and Vomiting**: Chemotherapy, in particular, is notorious for causing nausea and vomiting. This can lead to a reduced appetite and difficulty keeping food down.

2. **Mouth Sores**: Painful mouth sores, also known as mucositis, can develop due to chemotherapy and radiation therapy. These sores make eating and drinking painful and can lead to a decrease in food intake.

3. **Appetite Changes**: Some leukemia patients may experience changes in taste and smell perception, which can affect food preferences and appetite.

4. **Fatigue**: Cancer-related fatigue is a common side effect of leukemia and its treatment. It can lead to decreased energy levels, making meal preparation and eating a challenge.

5. **Diarrhea or Constipation**: Digestive issues, such as diarrhea or constipation, can result from chemotherapy or medications and can affect nutrient absorption.

6. **Weight Loss:** Unintentional weight loss can occur during treatment due to a combination of factors, including nausea, loss of appetite, and metabolic changes.

Dietary Strategies for Managing Side Effects

Nutrition can be a powerful ally in managing these side effects and maintaining your strength and well-being during leukemia treatment.

Let's explore specific dietary strategies for addressing some common side effects:

1. Nausea and Vomiting:

- **Small, Frequent Meals**: Eating small, frequent meals throughout the day can help prevent nausea. Try to eat something light every few hours rather than three large meals.
- **Ginger**: Ginger has anti-nausea properties. Consider ginger tea,

ginger candies, or adding ginger to your meals.

- **Avoid Strong Odors**: Strong smells can trigger nausea. Opt for bland, non-greasy foods and avoid cooking or eating in a confined space with strong odors.

- **Stay Hydrated**: Dehydration can worsen nausea. Sip clear fluids like water, herbal tea, or clear broths to stay hydrated.

2. Mouth Sores:

- **Soft, Cool Foods**: Opt for soft, cool foods that are gentle on your mouth. Yogurt, smoothies, mashed potatoes, and chilled soups are good choices.

- **Avoid Spicy or Acidic Foods**: Spices and acidic foods can further irritate mouth sores. Stick to mild, neutral flavors.

- **Rinse with Saltwater**: Gargling with a warm

saltwater solution can help soothe mouth sores.

3. Appetite Changes:

- **Experiment with Flavors**: Taste changes can make familiar foods unappealing. Experiment with different flavors and seasonings to find what appeals to you.

- **Stay Hydrated**: Sometimes, thirst can be mistaken for lack of appetite. Be sure to drink enough fluids.

- **Nutrient-Dense Choices**: Focus on nutrient-dense foods to maximize the nutritional value of your meals.

4. Fatigue:

- **Energy-Dense Foods**: Choose energy-dense foods to combat fatigue. These include nuts, seeds, avocado, and whole grains.
- **Stay Hydrated**: Dehydration can worsen fatigue. Keep a water

bottle nearby to ensure you're drinking enough fluids.

5. Digestive Issues:

- **Fiber Management**: If you're experiencing diarrhea, avoid high-fiber foods that can exacerbate the issue. On the other hand, if you're constipated, include more fiber-rich foods like whole grains, fruits, and vegetables.

- **Probiotics**: Probiotic-rich foods like yogurt can support digestive health and may help alleviate some gastrointestinal symptoms.

6. Weight Loss:

- **Nutrient-Dense Foods**: Prioritize nutrient-dense foods to ensure you're getting the most nutrition from your meals, even if your appetite is reduced.

- **Calorie-Dense Foods**: Incorporate calorie-dense foods like nuts, nut butter, and avocados to help maintain or regain lost weight.

Individualized Approach

Remember that the effectiveness of these dietary strategies can vary from person to person. It's crucial to work closely with your healthcare team and a registered dietitian who can tailor a plan to your specific needs. They can provide personalized recommendations based on your type of leukemia, treatment regimen, and any preexisting medical conditions.

Supplements and Nutrition Support

In some cases, your healthcare team may recommend nutritional supplements to address specific deficiencies or side effects. For instance, oral nutritional supplements, which are high in calories and nutrients, can be prescribed to help maintain or regain weight.

Hydration Matters

Proper hydration is essential during leukemia treatment, as dehydration can worsen side effects and impact overall well-being. If you struggle to drink enough water due to taste changes or nausea, consider these hydration strategies:

- Sip fluids slowly throughout the day.
- Try flavored water or water with a splash of fruit juice to make it more appealing.
- Use a straw or a sippy cup if it's more comfortable.
- Consume hydrating foods like watermelon, cucumber, and oranges.
- Discuss the possibility of intravenous (IV) fluids with your healthcare

team if dehydration becomes severe.

Emotional Support

Managing treatment side effects can be emotionally challenging. It's essential to seek emotional support, which can, in turn, positively influence your appetite and overall well-being. Consider joining support groups, seeking counseling, or engaging in relaxation techniques to help cope with the emotional aspects of treatment.

As you navigate the journey of leukemia treatment, remember that nutrition can be a vital tool in managing side effects and enhancing your overall quality of life. With the right guidance and a personalized approach, you can optimize your diet to support your body's resilience and maintain your strength during this challenging time.

CHAPTER 7

Maintaining Energy and Strength

In Chapter 7 of "Leukemia Nutrition: Nourishing Your Journey to Wellness," we delve into the crucial topic of maintaining energy and strength during leukemia treatment. Leukemia, like many cancers, can sap your energy and leave you feeling physically and mentally drained. In this chapter, we'll explore how proper nutrition can be a powerful tool in combating fatigue, enhancing your strength, and supporting your overall well-being.

The Challenge of Fatigue

Cancer-related fatigue is one of the most common and debilitating side effects experienced by leukemia patients. It goes beyond ordinary tiredness and can significantly impact your daily life, making even simple tasks feel like monumental challenges.

Understanding the factors contributing to cancer-related fatigue can help you address them effectively:

1. **Anemia**: Many leukemia patients experience anemia, which is a condition characterized by a low red blood cell count. Red blood cells carry oxygen to the body's tissues, and when their numbers are

low, it can lead to fatigue and weakness.

2. **Nutritional Deficiencies**: Cancer and its treatments can lead to nutritional deficiencies, such as low levels of iron, vitamin B12, and folate. These deficiencies can contribute to fatigue.

3. **Sleep Disturbances**: Pain, anxiety, and medication side effects can disrupt sleep patterns, leaving you

feeling chronically fatigued.

4. **Emotional Stress**: The emotional toll of leukemia and its treatment can be draining, leading to physical fatigue.

5. **Inactivity**: Fatigue can lead to a decrease in physical activity, which, in turn, can exacerbate feelings of weakness and tiredness.

Nutrition as a Source of Energy

Proper nutrition is an essential component of managing fatigue and maintaining energy and strength during leukemia treatment. Your diet plays a pivotal role in providing the necessary nutrients to combat the factors contributing to fatigue. Here are some key dietary strategies to help you stay energized:

1. Addressing Anemia:

- **Iron-Rich Foods**: If anemia is a concern, incorporate iron-rich foods into your diet. Good sources include lean meats, poultry, fish, beans, lentils, and fortified cereals.

- **Vitamin C**: Enhance iron absorption by consuming foods high in vitamin C alongside iron-rich foods. Citrus fruits, strawberries, and bell peppers are excellent choices.

- **Folate and Vitamin B12**: Include foods rich in folate (leafy greens, beans) and vitamin B12 (lean meats, fish, dairy) to support red blood cell production.

2. Combatting Nutritional Deficiencies:

- **Supplements**: In some cases, your healthcare team may recommend supplements to address specific deficiencies. It's crucial to work closely with them to determine if supplements are necessary and at what dosage.

- **Nutrient-Dense Foods**: Prioritize nutrient-dense foods in your diet to ensure you're getting a wide array of vitamins and minerals. This can help combat deficiencies and support overall health.

3. Improving Sleep Quality:

- **Caffeine and Timing**: Limit caffeine intake, especially in the afternoon and evening, as it can disrupt sleep. Opt for herbal teas or warm milk before bedtime.

- **Sleep Hygiene**: Create a sleep-conducive environment by keeping your bedroom dark, quiet, and cool. Establish a regular sleep schedule.

- **Relaxation Techniques**: Engage in

relaxation practices like deep breathing exercises, meditation, or gentle stretches to promote restful sleep.

4. Managing Emotional Stress:

- **Emotional Support**: Seek emotional support through counseling, support groups, or talking to a trusted friend or family member. Reducing emotional stress can improve overall well-being and energy levels.

- **Mindful Eating**: Practice mindful eating to reduce stress-related overeating or undereating. Pay attention to your body's hunger and fullness cues.

5. Maintaining Physical Activity:

- **Exercise as Able**: Engaging in gentle physical activity, as tolerated, can help combat fatigue and improve overall strength. Consult with your healthcare team to determine the appropriate level of activity for your condition.

- **Balanced Diet**: Ensure your diet provides enough calories and nutrients to support physical activity. Proper nutrition can help you get the most out of your exercise routine.

Meal Planning for Energy and Strength

Crafting meals that boost your energy and maintain your strength is essential during leukemia treatment. Here's how you can plan your meals to combat fatigue:

1. **Balanced Diet:** Maintain a balanced diet that includes carbohydrates, proteins, and healthy fats to provide sustained energy.

2. **Frequent Meals**: Eating small, frequent meals can help prevent energy crashes and maintain your strength throughout the day.

3. **Energy-Dense Foods**: Include energy-dense foods like nuts, seeds, and avocados to provide a quick source of energy.

4. **Protein**: Prioritize protein-rich foods to support muscle strength and repair.

5. **Hydration**: Stay well-hydrated, as dehydration can worsen fatigue. Sip fluids regularly, especially if you're experiencing nausea or diarrhea.

6. **Vitamins and Minerals**: Ensure your meals include a variety of fruits and vegetables to provide essential vitamins and minerals.

7. **Moderation**: Enjoy treats and less nutritious foods in moderation to

maintain a balanced diet while still satisfying cravings.

Supplements and Energy Boosters

In some cases, your healthcare team may recommend specific supplements or energy boosters to help combat fatigue. These may include:

- **Oral Nutritional Supplements**: These calorie- and nutrient-dense drinks or shakes can be prescribed to help you meet your nutritional needs and maintain or regain weight.

- **B Vitamins**: Vitamin B complex supplements can help combat fatigue and improve energy levels.

- **Caffeine**: In moderation, caffeine may provide a temporary energy boost, but it's essential not to rely on it excessively.

- **Adaptogens**: Certain herbs and supplements like ginseng and rhodiola may help combat fatigue and improve stamina, but always consult with your healthcare team before using them.

Gradual Changes

It's important to make gradual dietary changes and not to overwhelm yourself with a complete overhaul of your eating habits, especially if you're already dealing with fatigue and other side effects. Small, sustainable changes can make a significant difference over time.

Final Thoughts

Chapter 7 underscores the pivotal role of nutrition in combating cancer-related fatigue and maintaining energy and strength during leukemia treatment. By understanding the factors contributing to fatigue and implementing dietary strategies tailored to your needs, you can enhance your overall well-being and better navigate the challenges of leukemia. Remember to work closely with your healthcare team and a registered dietitian to ensure that your nutrition plan aligns with your specific condition and treatment.

CHAPTER 8

Promoting Emotional Well-Being

In Chapter 8 of "Leukemia Nutrition: Nourishing Your Journey to Wellness," we delve into the profound connection between nutrition and emotional well-being during your leukemia journey. Facing a leukemia diagnosis and undergoing treatment can be emotionally challenging, and your diet can play a vital role in supporting your mental and emotional health. This chapter explores the impact of nutrition on mood and offers strategies to promote emotional well-being.

The Mind-Body Connection

The link between nutrition and emotional well-being is a growing area of research. Emerging evidence suggests that what you eat can significantly influence your mood and mental health. Here are some key aspects of this mind-body connection:

1. **Nutrient Deficiencies and Mood**: Nutrient deficiencies, such as low levels of certain vitamins and minerals, can contribute to mood disturbances, including anxiety and depression. For example, low levels of vitamin D and folate have been associated

with an increased risk of depression.

2. **Gut-Brain Axis**: The gut and brain are intricately connected through the gut-brain axis. The gut microbiome, which is influenced by your diet, can affect mood and mental health. A healthy gut microbiome is associated with improved mood and reduced risk of mood disorders.

3. **Inflammation**: Chronic inflammation, often linked to poor dietary choices, has been implicated in the development of mood disorders. A diet high in processed foods, sugar, and unhealthy fats can promote inflammation, while a diet rich in fruits, vegetables, and anti-inflammatory foods can help reduce it.

Strategies for Promoting Emotional Well-Being Through Nutrition

Now, let's explore practical strategies for promoting emotional well-being through your diet during your leukemia journey:

1. Focus on Whole Foods:

- **Fruits and Vegetables**: Incorporate a variety of colorful fruits and vegetables into your meals. They are rich in vitamins, minerals, and antioxidants that support mental health.

- **Whole Grains**: Opt for whole grains like brown rice, quinoa, and whole wheat bread instead of refined grains. These provide sustained energy and help stabilize mood.

- **Lean Proteins**: Choose lean sources of protein such as poultry, fish, beans, and tofu. Protein contains amino acids that are essential for neurotransmitter production, which can influence mood.

2. Omega-3 Fatty Acids:

- **Fatty Fish**: Include fatty fish like salmon, mackerel, and sardines in your diet. They are rich in omega-3 fatty acids, which have been linked to improved mood and reduced risk of depression.

- **Flaxseeds and Walnuts**: If you don't consume fish, consider flaxseeds and walnuts as plant-based sources of omega-3s.

3. Probiotics and Gut Health:

- **Yogurt and Fermented Foods**: Incorporate yogurt with live cultures, kefir, sauerkraut, and other fermented foods into your diet. These can help promote a healthy gut microbiome, which may support better mood.

4. Nutrient-Rich Snacks:

- **Nuts and Seeds**: Snack on nuts and seeds like almonds, sunflower seeds, and pumpkin seeds. They provide healthy fats, protein, and nutrients that can help stabilize blood sugar levels and prevent mood swings.

- **Fruit with Nut Butter**: Pair sliced apples or bananas with nut butter for a satisfying and nutrient-rich snack.

5. Hydration:

- **Water**: Dehydration can affect mood and cognitive function. Be sure to stay adequately hydrated by drinking water throughout the day.

6. Limit Sugar and Processed Foods:

- **Sugar**: Minimize the consumption of sugary foods and beverages. Excess sugar can lead to energy fluctuations and worsen mood swings.

- **Processed Foods**: Highly processed foods often contain unhealthy fats and additives that can negatively impact mood. Choose whole, minimally processed foods whenever possible.

7. Balanced Meals:

- **Regular Eating Schedule**: Maintain a regular eating schedule to prevent fluctuations in blood sugar levels, which can affect mood and energy levels.

- **Balanced Macronutrients**: Include a balance of carbohydrates, proteins, and healthy fats in your meals to provide sustained energy and stabilize mood.

8. Mindful Eating:

- **Eat Mindfully**: Pay attention to your mealtime experience. Savor the flavors, textures, and aromas of your food. Eating mindfully can enhance the pleasure of eating and promote a positive relationship with food.

9. Seek Professional Guidance:

- **Registered Dietitian**: If you're struggling with mood disturbances or emotional challenges, consider working with a registered dietitian who specializes in nutrition and mental health. They can provide personalized guidance and support.

10. Emotional Support:

- **Support Groups**: Consider joining support groups or seeking counseling to address emotional challenges related to your leukemia diagnosis and treatment. Emotional support is a crucial component of overall well-being.

Moderation and Balance

While nutrition can significantly influence emotional well-being, it's essential to maintain a balanced and realistic approach to diet. Strive for moderation rather than perfection. Enjoy treats and less nutritious foods in moderation, and don't be too hard on yourself if your diet isn't flawless. The goal is to create a nourishing and sustainable relationship with food that supports your emotional well-being.

Conclusion

Chapter 8 underscores the vital connection between

nutrition and emotional well-being during your leukemia journey. By making thoughtful dietary choices and prioritizing nutrient-rich foods, you can promote better mood, reduce the risk of mood disturbances, and support your overall mental health. Remember that seeking professional guidance and emotional support when needed is an essential aspect of your holistic well-being as you navigate the emotional challenges of leukemia and its treatment.

CHAPTER 9

Coping with Dietary Challenges and Special Situations

Chapter 9 of "Leukemia Nutrition: Nourishing Your Journey to Wellness" addresses the various dietary challenges and special situations that leukemia patients may encounter during their treatment and recovery. Leukemia treatment can bring about a range of unique circumstances, from dietary restrictions to specific symptoms that require tailored nutrition strategies. This chapter provides guidance on navigating these challenges to ensure you continue to receive the nourishment your body needs.

Dietary Challenges and Special Situations

Leukemia patients often face distinct dietary challenges and special situations that can impact their nutrition. Here are some of the key scenarios explored in this chapter:

1. Dietary Restrictions:

- **Blood-Thinning Medications**: Some leukemia patients may be prescribed blood-thinning medications, which can require dietary adjustments to manage vitamin K intake. This vitamin plays a role in blood clotting, and its consumption must be consistent.

- **Infection Precautions**: During treatment, leukemia patients are more vulnerable to infections due to compromised immune systems. This may necessitate dietary precautions to reduce the risk of foodborne illnesses.

2. Gastrointestinal Symptoms:

- **Nausea and Vomiting**: Ongoing or treatment-induced nausea and vomiting can make eating challenging. Coping strategies include consuming small, bland meals, staying hydrated, and working with healthcare professionals to manage these symptoms.

- **Diarrhea or Constipation**: Gastrointestinal symptoms like diarrhea or constipation can disrupt normal eating patterns. Tailoring your diet to address these issues involves adjusting fiber intake and staying well-hydrated.

3. Swallowing Difficulties:

- **Dysphagia**: Some leukemia patients may experience difficulty swallowing (dysphagia), which can limit food choices. Pureed or soft-textured foods, thickened liquids, and swallowing exercises may be necessary.

4. Oral Health Challenges:

- **Mouth Sores (Mucositis)**: Painful mouth sores can make eating and drinking uncomfortable. Soft, cool, and bland foods are often recommended to soothe these sores.

- **Dry Mouth (Xerostomia)**: Dry mouth can affect taste

and make eating difficult. Staying hydrated and using sugar-free gum or lozenges can help manage this symptom.

5. Nutritional Support:

- **Enteral Nutrition**: In some cases, when eating is not possible or sufficient, enteral nutrition (feeding through a tube) may be required to ensure adequate nutrition.

- **Parenteral Nutrition**: Parenteral nutrition, which involves intravenous delivery of nutrients, may be necessary when the gastrointestinal tract cannot be used for nutrition.

Tailoring Your Diet to Special Situations

Navigating these dietary challenges and special situations requires a tailored approach. Here are strategies for coping with each scenario:

1. Blood-Thinning Medications:

- **Consistent Vitamin K Intake**: If you're on blood-thinning medications like warfarin, work with a healthcare professional to maintain consistent vitamin K intake from foods like leafy greens, broccoli, and Brussels sprouts.

2. Infection Precautions:

- **Safe Food Handling**: Follow food safety practices, such as thoroughly cooking meats, washing fruits and vegetables, and avoiding raw or undercooked eggs and seafood.

- **Hydration**: Stay well-hydrated to support overall health and immune function.

3.   Gastrointestinal Symptoms:

- **Nausea and Vomiting**: Opt for small, frequent meals with mild flavors. Stay hydrated with clear fluids, and consider ginger and other nausea-reducing remedies.

- **Diarrhea or Constipation**: Adjust your fiber intake based on your symptoms. For diarrhea, opt for low-fiber, easily digestible foods. For constipation, incorporate more high-fiber foods like whole grains, fruits, and vegetables.

4. Swallowing Difficulties:

- **Texture Modifications**: If you have difficulty swallowing, work with a dietitian to develop a diet plan that includes pureed or soft-textured foods that are easier to swallow.

5. Oral Health Challenges:

- **Mouth Sores (Mucositis)**: Choose cool, soft, and bland foods that are gentle on the mouth. Avoid spicy, acidic, or rough-textured foods.

- **Dry Mouth (Xerostomia)**: Sip water throughout the day and use sugar-free gum or lozenges to help stimulate saliva production.

6. Nutritional Support:

- **Enteral Nutrition**: If enteral nutrition is necessary, work with a registered dietitian to develop a feeding plan tailored to your needs and preferences.

- **Parenteral Nutrition**: Parenteral nutrition is typically administered in a hospital or clinical setting. Your healthcare team will closely monitor your nutritional needs and make adjustments as needed.

Personalized Guidance is Key

The key to successfully coping with these dietary challenges and special situations is personalized guidance. A registered dietitian with experience in oncology nutrition can provide invaluable support in developing a tailored nutrition plan that addresses your unique circumstances.

Emotional and Psychological Impact

Beyond the physical challenges, it's essential to recognize the emotional and psychological impact of these dietary challenges. Coping with dietary restrictions, symptoms, or medical interventions can be emotionally taxing. Seek emotional support through counseling, support groups, or talking to a trusted friend or family member to help navigate the emotional aspects of these situations.

Maintaining a Positive Outlook

Coping with dietary challenges and special situations during leukemia treatment can be daunting, but it's important to maintain a positive outlook. Remember that your healthcare team is there to provide guidance and support, and there are resources available to help you adapt to these circumstances. By working closely with your healthcare providers and a registered dietitian, you can find solutions that allow you to continue receiving the nourishment your body needs to support your health and well-being.

Conclusion

Chapter 9 acknowledges the various dietary challenges and special situations that leukemia patients may encounter during their journey. By tailoring your diet to address these unique circumstances and seeking personalized guidance from healthcare professionals, you can continue to nourish your body and maintain your strength and resilience. Remember that emotional support is equally important in managing the emotional impact of these challenges, so don't hesitate to seek help when needed. Your well-being is a holistic endeavor, and nutrition plays a crucial role in supporting it.

CHAPTER 10

Long-Term Nutrition and Wellness

In the final chapter of "Leukemia Nutrition: Nourishing Your Journey to Wellness," we delve into the critical topic of long-term nutrition and wellness for leukemia survivors. Beyond the active phase of treatment, maintaining a healthy and balanced diet remains crucial to support your overall well-being, reduce the risk of complications, and enhance your quality of life. This chapter explores the challenges and strategies for long-term nutrition and wellness after leukemia treatment.

Transitioning to Life After Treatment

Surviving leukemia is a significant accomplishment, but it often marks the beginning of a new chapter filled with adjustments and uncertainties. Transitioning from active treatment to life after leukemia can be both exciting and challenging. Here are some key considerations:

1. Monitoring and Follow-Up Care:

- Regular medical check-ups and follow-up appointments with your oncologist are essential to monitor for any signs of leukemia recurrence or potential late effects of treatment.

- Blood tests and imaging may be part of these follow-up appointments to ensure your health and well-being.

2.   Emotional and Psychological Well-Being:

- Coping with the emotional aftermath of leukemia and treatment is an ongoing process. Seek emotional support through counseling, support groups, or therapy to help you navigate the psychological impact of your experience.

3. Managing Late Effects:

- Some leukemia survivors may experience late effects of treatment, which can include cardiovascular issues, bone health problems, and fertility concerns, among others.

- It's essential to address these late effects with your healthcare team and work together to develop strategies for managing them.

4. Lifestyle and Wellness:

- Focus on lifestyle choices that promote overall well-being, including regular exercise, stress management, and adequate sleep.

- Nutrition plays a vital role in supporting these

aspects of wellness and helping you lead a fulfilling life after leukemia.

Challenges in Long-Term Nutrition and Wellness

As a leukemia survivor, you may encounter specific challenges related to nutrition and wellness. These can include:

1. Maintaining a Balanced Diet:

- After treatment, it's important to continue consuming a balanced diet that provides essential nutrients to support your overall health. A balanced diet includes a variety of fruits, vegetables, lean proteins, whole grains, and healthy fats.

- Nutrient deficiencies, which can result from treatment or dietary restrictions, should be addressed through careful meal planning and, if necessary, supplements.

2. Staying Physically Active:

- Regular physical activity is crucial for maintaining a healthy weight, promoting cardiovascular health, and reducing the risk of certain late effects of treatment.

- Leukemia survivors should aim for at least

150 minutes of moderate-intensity exercise or 75 minutes of vigorous-intensity exercise per week, as recommended by health guidelines.

3. Managing Weight and Body Composition:

- Some survivors may experience weight changes, either as a result of treatment or lifestyle factors.

- Maintaining a healthy weight is essential for reducing the risk of certain health complications, such as cardiovascular disease and diabetes.

4. Emotional Eating and Stress:

- Coping with the emotional aftermath of leukemia can sometimes lead to emotional eating or stress-induced eating habits.

- It's important to be mindful of emotional eating patterns and seek healthier ways to manage stress and emotions, such as through relaxation techniques, therapy, or support groups.

Strategies for Long-Term Nutrition and Wellness

To navigate the challenges of long-term nutrition and wellness after leukemia, consider these strategies:

1.   **Maintain   Regular Follow-Up Care:**

- Continue with regular medical check-ups and follow-up appointments to monitor your health and detect any potential issues early.

2. **Create a Sustainable Diet Plan:**

- Work with a registered dietitian to develop a sustainable, long-term diet plan that aligns with your health goals and addresses any specific dietary concerns.

3. Prioritize Nutrient-Rich Foods:

- Continue to prioritize nutrient-dense foods in your diet, including fruits, vegetables, whole grains, lean proteins, and healthy fats.

4. Monitor and Manage Weight:

- If weight management is a concern, consider working with a healthcare professional or dietitian to establish a healthy weight management plan that includes balanced nutrition and regular physical activity.

5. Stay Active:

- Incorporate regular physical activity into your routine. Find activities you enjoy to make exercise a sustainable part of your lifestyle.

6. Stress Management:

- Practice stress management techniques, such as mindfulness, meditation, or deep breathing exercises, to help you cope with the emotional aspects of your journey.

7. Emotional Support:

- Continue seeking emotional support as needed, whether through therapy, support groups, or counseling. Emotional well-being is an integral part of your overall health.

8. Communicate with Your Healthcare Team:

- Maintain open communication with your healthcare team about any health concerns or late effects of treatment that may arise.

9. Be Adaptable:

- Be open to adapting your diet and lifestyle as needed to accommodate any changes in your health or well-being.

10. Set Realistic Goals:

vbnet

- Set achievable goals for your nutrition, fitness, and overall wellness. It's important to be patient with yourself and celebrate your progress along the way.

Conclusion

Chapter 10 emphasizes the importance of long-term nutrition and wellness for leukemia survivors. While completing treatment is a significant milestone, maintaining your health and well-being is an ongoing journey. By staying engaged in your medical care, making informed choices about your diet and lifestyle, and seeking support when needed, you can continue to thrive and lead a fulfilling life after leukemia. Remember that you are not alone in this journey, and your healthcare team, along with a network of support, is there to guide you every step of the way.

CHAPTER 11

Building a Sustainable Future

In the concluding chapter of "Leukemia Nutrition: Nourishing Your Journey to Wellness," we explore the concept of building a sustainable future after leukemia. This chapter focuses on how to maintain the progress made in terms of nutrition, wellness, and overall well-being while looking ahead to a brighter and more resilient future.

The Journey Towards Sustainability

Surviving leukemia is a remarkable achievement, and it signifies a new beginning filled with hope and opportunities. However, the journey towards sustainability, both in terms of health and well-being, requires careful planning and a proactive approach. Here are some key elements to consider:

1.   **Wellness Beyond Treatment:**

- Your journey continues beyond the active phase of leukemia treatment. Transitioning to a wellness-focused approach involves taking the lessons learned during treatment and applying them to a long-term health and well-being plan.

2. Nutrition as a Lifestyle:

- Nutrition isn't just about following a diet during treatment; it's about making sustainable, healthy choices that support your well-being over the long term.

- Embrace nutrition as a lifestyle, incorporating nourishing foods into your daily routine.

3. Physical Activity and Fitness:

- Regular physical activity is a cornerstone of a sustainable future. It helps maintain a healthy weight, supports cardiovascular health, and reduces the risk of late effects of treatment.

- Aim to find activities you enjoy to ensure that exercise becomes a sustainable part of your life.

4. Emotional Resilience:

- Emotional well-being is a critical component of sustainability. Building emotional resilience involves managing stress, seeking support when needed, and cultivating a positive outlook on life.

5. Setting and Achieving Goals:

- Set realistic goals for your health and wellness journey. These can include nutritional goals, fitness milestones, and emotional well-being objectives.

- Celebrate your achievements along the way, no matter how small they may seem.

Sustainability Challenges and Strategies

Building a sustainable future after leukemia comes with its own set of challenges. Let's explore these challenges and the strategies to overcome them:

1. Fear of Recurrence:

- One of the most significant challenges leukemia survivors face is the fear of recurrence. This fear can be overwhelming and impact your emotional well-being.

- Strategies for coping with this fear include regular follow-up appointments with your healthcare team, engaging in stress-reducing practices, and seeking support from a therapist or support group.

2. Lifestyle Changes:

- Transitioning to a healthier lifestyle can be challenging, especially if you were not accustomed to it before your leukemia diagnosis.

- Begin with small, sustainable changes in your diet and exercise routine. Gradual adjustments are more likely to stick in the long run.

3. Finding Motivation:

- Maintaining motivation for sustained wellness can be difficult. Motivation often wanes over time.
- Stay motivated by setting clear goals, tracking your progress, and rewarding yourself for achievements.

4. Busy Life and Time Constraints:

- A busy lifestyle can make it challenging to prioritize nutrition and wellness.

- Plan and schedule your meals and exercise like you would any other important appointment. Time management and prioritization are key.

5. Social and Peer Pressure:

- Social situations and peer pressure can sometimes lead to unhealthy choices, such as overindulging in unhealthy foods or skipping workouts.

- Communicate your goals and priorities to friends and family, and seek their support in maintaining a healthy lifestyle.

Strategies for a Sustainable Future

Here are strategies to help you build a sustainable future after leukemia:

1. Develop a Wellness Plan:

- Work with your healthcare team, including a registered dietitian and fitness professional, to develop a personalized wellness plan. This plan should include nutrition, exercise, and emotional well-being components.

2. Establish Healthy Habits:

- Gradually incorporate healthy habits into your daily life, such as making balanced food choices, staying active, and practicing stress-reduction techniques.

3. Prioritize Self-Care:

- Self-care is vital for sustainability. Make time for self-care activities that rejuvenate and relax you, whether it's reading, taking nature walks, or engaging in hobbies.

4. Build a Support System:

- Surround yourself with a supportive network of friends and family who understand your goals and encourage your efforts.

- Consider joining a support group for leukemia survivors to connect with others who

share   similar
experiences.

5. Set SMART Goals:

- SMART goals are Specific, Measurable, Achievable, Relevant, and Time-bound. These types of goals are more likely to be achieved and provide a sense of accomplishment.

6. Celebrate Successes:

- Celebrate your achievements, no matter

how small they may seem. Acknowledging your progress can boost motivation and confidence.

7. Monitor and Adjust:

- Regularly assess your wellness plan and make adjustments as needed. Your needs and circumstances may change over time, and your plan should reflect that.

Conclusion

Chapter 11 highlights the concept of building a sustainable future after leukemia. While the journey through leukemia treatment is undoubtedly challenging, it can also be transformative. By applying the lessons learned, adopting a holistic approach to health and well-being, and setting realistic goals, you can embark on a journey of sustainability and resilience. Remember that you are not alone in this journey; your healthcare team, support network, and your inner strength will guide you toward a future filled with health, happiness, and fulfillment. Your experience with leukemia has equipped you with a unique perspective on life, and with the right strategies, you can create a sustainable future filled with vitality and purpose.

CONCLUSION

In closing, "Leukemia Nutrition: Nourishing Your Journey to Wellness" has taken us on a profound expedition through the crucial role of nutrition in the lives of leukemia patients and survivors. We've journeyed through 11 chapters that have explored not only the science behind leukemia nutrition but also the deeply human aspects of coping, healing, and thriving. As we conclude this odyssey, let's reflect on the transformative power of knowledge, support, and resilience that this book has illuminated.

The pages of this book have been filled with insights, strategies, and guidance that extend far beyond dietary choices. We've explored the physical, emotional, and psychological dimensions of the leukemia journey, recognizing that health and wellness are not confined to what we eat but encompass our entire well-being. The lessons learned can be summarized in three key takeaways:

1.   Knowledge is Empowerment:

- Understanding the profound relationship between nutrition and leukemia is the first step towards empowerment. Armed with knowledge, patients and caregivers can make informed decisions about their diet, lifestyle, and treatment.

- Through each chapter, we've unearthed the nutritional tools and strategies that can enhance resilience, alleviate side effects, and support overall health. From managing fatigue to promoting emotional well-being, these insights are the lanterns that guide us through the darkest times.

2. Support is Invaluable:

- No one should navigate the labyrinth of leukemia alone. Support, whether from healthcare professionals, friends, family, or support groups, is a beacon of strength.

- This book has emphasized the importance of seeking emotional, nutritional, and medical support. Just as nutrition is a holistic endeavor, so is our well-being. Leukemia teaches us that vulnerability is not a weakness, but a bridge to connection and healing.

3. Resilience is the Truest Treasure:

- The journey through leukemia is a testament to the extraordinary resilience of the human spirit. It is a reminder that within each of us lies the power to overcome adversity, adapt to change, and embrace life with newfound appreciation.

- The stories of survivors and the wisdom shared in these chapters echo the unwavering resilience that defines the human experience. Through the darkest storms, we can discover our inner strength, transforming challenges into opportunities for growth and renewal.

As we reach the end of this journey, remember that the path to wellness is not a straight line; it's a dynamic and ever-evolving process. What we've learned in these pages is a foundation upon which you can continue to build a life of vitality and purpose.

Whether you are a leukemia patient, a caregiver, or simply someone seeking a deeper understanding of nutrition and well-being, the lessons of this book extend far beyond the realm of leukemia. They are universal truths that remind us of the incredible capacity of the human spirit to heal, adapt, and thrive.

So, as you turn the final page of "Leukemia Nutrition: Nourishing Your Journey to Wellness," carry forward the knowledge, support, and resilience you've discovered. Let it guide you not only in the face of adversity but also in your pursuit of a life that is nourished, whole, and sustainable. Your journey continues, and with each step, you are moving towards a brighter and more resilient future.

www.ingramcontent.com/pod-product-compliance
Lightning Source LLC
Chambersburg PA
CBHW050907260726
48660CB00001B/75

9 798866 462964